KETO BREAD COOKBOOK 2018

40 LOW CARB BREAD RECIPES FOR FAST KETOSIS, FAT BURNING & WEIGHT LOSS (INCLUDES NUTRITIONAL INFO, KETOGENIC BEGINNERS GUIDE, LOAVES, BREAD, BAGEL, SNACK RECIPES & MORE)

MEGAN O'NEIL

Copyright © 2018 by Christopher Raymont. All Right Reserved.

No part of this publication may be reproduced, distributed, or transmitted in any form or by any means, including photocopying, recording, or other electronic or mechanical methods, or by any information storage and retrieval system without the prior written permission of the publisher, except in the case of very brief quotations embodied in critical reviews and certain other noncommercial uses permitted by copyright law.

Contents

WELCOME TO THE KETO BREAD COOKBOOK

Hello and welcome to The Keto bread Cookbook 2019. Committing to a keto friendly diet usually means 2 things. And those two things are reducing your carb intake and increasing your fat intake. However, finding foods that are low in carbs and high in fat can be quite the effort. We should already know that in order to enter a state of ketosis, we need to have both components in our diet working correctly.

And that's exactly where keto bread comes into play. Inside this cookbook we shall look at what keto bread is, how it can help us reach ketosis and then look at some mouth-watering recipes that you can make.

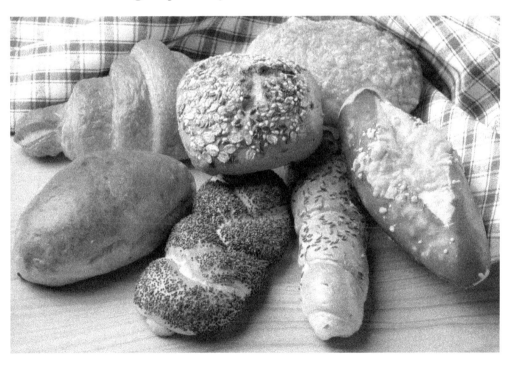

A BRIEFING ON KETO BREAD

Keto bread is great. Fact. However, from what I've seen, it's not much of a big deal in the keto industry now. And that's a great shame as some of the bread recipes you can make are far tastier and more exciting than carb-bread.

Traditional bread is awful. Carb content in your typical loaf of bread is incredibly high, which is possibly the worst food you can eat when following a ketogenic diet. With our keto-friendly bread recipes, each one of them is made up of less than 10 grams of carbs, ensuring that you stay in ketosis.

Keto bread can be enjoyed with a huge variety of toppings and used as a side dish and even as an appetite suppressing snack! With a huge variety of recipes in this book, you'll likely find your 'go to' favorites and more than likely enjoy each and every recipe you try.

Inside this cookbook you will not only discover your traditional loaf-type recipes, but also a whole host of exciting recipes you may have never even heard of before! You may have noticed there are a few fruit-based recipes included, but please don't panic! The sugar content in berries is generally very low and really won't make any difference to your state of ketosis.

BENEFITS OF EATING KETO BREAD

Before we get into the recipe side of the book, let's get our motivation levels up by taking a quick look at some of the benefits to adding keto bread to your diet!

High fat – While you probably won't want to try and get all your fat intake from keto bread, it remains a decent source of fat for your ketogenic needs.

Low carb – And this goes without saying, as per any recipe in your keto arsenal, that the carb content in our keto bread is VERY low, so you don't have to worry about suffering from carb crashes.

Easy to make – Lifestyles can be hectic, and not many of us have time to spend hours slaving away in the kitchen to pursue our health requirements. Our keto bread recipes are very simply, easy to follow, and won't have you worrying about time.

So much variety – There's no need to get bored and give up on your diet anymore. With these 40 recipes, you'll surely never get bored of eating keto bread.

Great taste – While great taste is obviously very subjective, I've personally found my pallet to adjust to keto bread recipes very nicely, and there's no looking back to high carb bread for me. Give all the recipes a try and you'll be surprised how quickly you adjust!

So, that's keto bread covered. Let's look now at the ketogenic diet before we move on to the recipes.

WHAT IS A KETOGENIC (KETO) DIET?

The ketogenic diet is a high-fat, medium protein, low-carb diet which has been making waves in the diet world. What captures the attention of people towards this diet is its effectiveness towards weight loss and preventing other health issues while enjoying tasty wholesome high-fat food.

In the ketogenic diet, 75% of calories should come from fat, 25% from proteins and 5% from carbohydrates. Making the body enter a metabolic state of ketosis is what the ketogenic diet aims to achieve. Carbohydrates are the body's primary choice over other fuel sources. So, when there is a lack of carbohydrates in the body, the body considers itself in diet mode.

This results in fat entering the blood, which in turn helps to create new roadways for the cells to get new sources of energy. Insulin is one of the body's main fat storing hormone. Due to reduced carb intake and increased usage of fat, the level of glucose and insulin in the bloodstream decreases.

One of these alternate pathways created during this process is ketogenesis and the result of ketogenesis is the production of ketone bodies. Ketones are produced when the liver breaks down fat which then become the body's primary source of energy. Ketones are a better source of energy and can even help in protecting brain cells when burned.

This is especially true when compared to the burning of carbohydrates, which create oxidative cells that cause damage and inflammation of cells when accumulated in huge amounts. This is the reason why people should avoid taking in more sugar than what is necessary.

Before starting the ketogenic diet, it is always advisable to consult your physician as drastic changes in diet can cause health issues in certain people because of their health conditions.

BENEFITS OF A KETOGENIC DIET

Controversy has always surrounded low carb diets and the effects on the body. However, there have been plenty of human studies conducted using low carb diets that have produced very promising outcomes.

Here are just a few of the reported benefits.

Weight loss – quite possibly the number one reason people start following the keto diet, is weight loss. Not only does voiding your body of carbs help you burn off fat, but you'll also be eating foods that are much lower in calories, which is equally as important for weight loss.

Appetite suppression – pretty important when dieting. Hunger can be an absolute nightmare, and often leads to binging on junk food. When we cut carbs from our body, we tend to replace them with foods high in protein and fat, which in turn leads to feeling much more satisfied while consuming less.

Reduced blood sugar and insulin levels – After eating carbohydrates, they break down inside our body into 'simple sugars' inside our digestive tract. This causes a rise in blood sugar levels when they enter the bloodstream. High blood sugars are toxic and cause your body to produce a hormone called insulin. Insulin 'tells' your body it's time to bring the simple sugars into our cells to either store them or burn them off.

A lot of people have a problem with this process, where it's harder for the body to bring blood sugar into cells. This ultimately can lead to type 2 diabetes.

By cutting out carbs, or following a ketogenic diet, you remove any need for insulin, which in turn solves this issue that at least 300 million people suffer from.

Blood pressure can go down – high blood pressure can bring about many diseases later in life, including heart disease. A low-carb or keto diet has been proven to help lower your blood pressure as thus lessen the risk of diseases.

More energy – During ketosis, your body uses fat as an energy source that will ultimately never run out, which means you'll find that you have a lot more energy during the day, and even enjoy a lifestyle that doesn't involve craving midday naps.

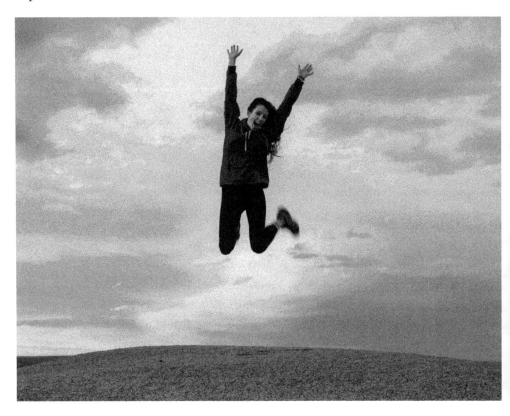

FOODS TO AVOID ON KETO

The following lists are going to be an absolute Godsend when it comes to starting your new diet. Let's look at the main culprits when it comes to slowing down your keto progressions.

Sugar – quite possibly the biggest no-no on the list. Unfortunately, sugar is found in a hell of a lot of foods these days. This is usually what people struggle to reduce the most in their diets.

Sugar is found in candy, cookies, chocolate, donuts, ice cream, cereals, milk, vitamin water, cakes and pretty much any other 'unhealthy' food that comes to mind.

Please bear in mind that the keto diet doesn't mean that you must have ZERO sugar per day. It's in almost everything we eat and won't be avoided. You need to think more so about the ADDITIONAL sugar that's getting added to your diet. Some of my recipes have TINY amounts of sugar in them that you can easily fit into your macros. Just be careful with it.

Starches – all the 'carby' foods you can think of are at risk of slowing your keto diet down. These include rice, bread and pasta as the obvious trio.

Beer – sorry to say that beer is full of carbs and will have to be limited on your new diet. There are some lower-carb beers that do exist if you crave it.

Fruit – not as bad as it is typically seen as a health food – however, fruits are indeed packed with sugar and should be limited on a keto diet. Berries, however, are typically low in sugar and fine to consume in moderation!

Please note again: you shouldn't mistake the keto diet as a NO CARB diet, when, it's a LOW CARB one. As a rough guide to how many carbs you can allow in your diet, you'll want to look between 20 and 50 grams per day. Obviously the closer to 20 grams you get, the more success you'll have.

With that briefing in mind, here's a list I've created that outlines over 100 foods you may want to avoid when going keto.

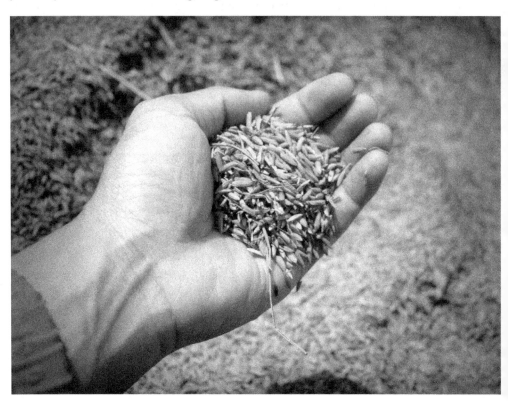

100+ Foods To Avoid on Keto

Grains: Wheat, oats, barley, rice, rye, corn, quinoa, millet, sorghum, bulgur, amaranth, sprouted grains, buckwheat. Any breads and pastas made from these foods also.

Beans and legumes: Kidney beans, chickpeas, black beans, lentils, green peas, lima beans, pinto beans, white beans, cannellini beans, fava beans, black-eyed beans

Fruits: Bananas, pineapples, apples, papaya, grapes, oranges, mangos, tangerines, fruit juices, smoothies, dried fruits, fruit syrups, fruit concentrates

Vegetables: Yams, sweet potatoes, carrots, parsnips, peas, yucca, corn, cherry tomatoes

Sugars: Honey, agave nectar, maple syrup, raw sugar, cane sugar, high-fructose corn syrup, turbinado sugar

Protein: Milk, butter substitutes, cream cheese, evaporated milk, whipped topping, low-fat yogurts

Fats: Soybean oil, peanut oil, sesame oil, sunflower oil, safflower oil, grapeseed oil, corn oil, canola oil

Drinks: Beer, wines, cocktails, mixers, flavored liquors, sodas, diet sodas, fruit juice, smoothies, coffee/tea with added sweetener, sweetened milk products

THE BREAKDOWN

With the above lists in mind, let's look at what kind of percentages you want to aim for with your macronutrients to stay in a ketosis state.

Carbs: As we already know, the keto diet is heavily based on reducing carbs, therefore we want to look at carbs making up around **5-10%** of our daily intake of food.

Fat: Now our primary source of energy, we want to start upping the fat intake in our diet. We need our fat intake to take up around **70-80%** of our daily intake.

Protein: Unless you're looking to win the next Mr. Olympia, you don't need to worry about consuming too much protein. A moderate amount of around **20-25%** each day should suffice.

This doesn't mean that you must stick EXACTLY to the numbers and foods recommended in this book, however, just be aware that swaying off course too often will take you out of a ketosis state and reverse the progress – try your best to cut the foods out of your diet I've listed and stick to the percentages above.

QUICK TIPS FOR KETO DIET SUCCESS

Quick tips are great for lazy people like me who don't want to learn all the 'sciencey' malarkey that goes behind certain diets. Let's look at my top tips for success with the keto diet.

Stop eating out – eating out regularly at restaurants or takeaways is the easiest way to ruin your keto diet. Restaurant and takeaway foods are PACKED full of calories and carbs. The problem with this type of food is that it's not immediately obvious what you are consuming. The bulk of your food should come from homemade recipes!

If it's in the house, you'll eat it – quite possibly my favorite tip in this list. It may seem obvious, but it works very well. Don't stock your cabinets full of foods you know you shouldn't have. If they exist in the house, chances are at some point you will consume it, so don't buy the food in the first place. Stay strong.

Look at what you're eating – again, look at what you're eating. Check the packs of the food for carbs and make sure they fit into your daily allowance of carbohydrates.

Social support – the keto diet has now become so popular that you are never going to be alone with your quest for superior health. There are now hundreds of forums and groups online you can join and participate in. These are extremely handy for when you have questions or just want some support when getting started.

Be prepared for changes – when switching diets, your body goes through a lot of changes and you need to be mentally prepared for this to potentially happen when going low-carb. During your first few days of keto, you may experience some flu-like symptoms. Just make sure you drink plenty of water and healthy foods – it will pass. Always get seen to by a doctor if you're unsure.

Meal prep if you can – preparing your meals for the entire week is a great way to ensure you stick to your new diet. Trying to take your diet as and when it comes almost nearly always ends up in binge eating. Fail to plan, plan to fail!

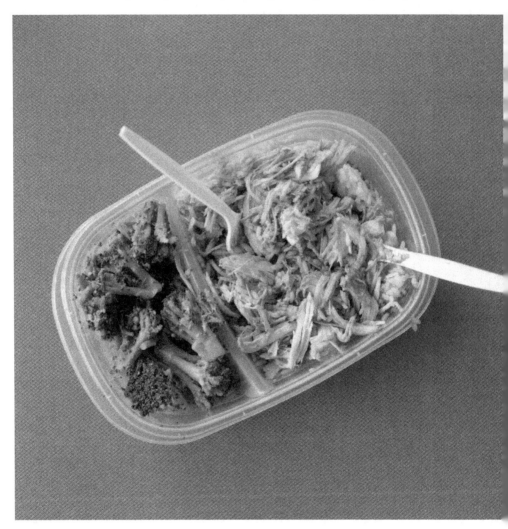

LOW CARB CHEAT LIST

We've already looked at what we can't eat, so let's now look at what we can eat. I've created this cheat list of low carb foods, so you can refer to it at any given point for help when creating meals or snacking.

Replace flavored yogurt with: coconut milk yogurt, sour cream, full fat cottage cheese, full fat Greek yogurt

Replace cereals with: Salted caramel pork rind cereal, toasted nuts, flax granola, chia pudding

Replace oatmeal with: Cinnamon roll oatmeal, cauliflower, chia seed, flax meal oatmeal

Replace pancakes and waffles with: Peanut butter pancakes, cream cheese pancakes, almond flour waffles

Replaces egg whites: Whole eggs

Replace burger and fries: Steak and vegetables, burger with no bun

Replace typical pizza: Mozzarella cheese dough pizza, pizza casserole

Replace bread crust fried chicken with: Pork Rind and Parmesan crust

Replace processed soups with: Pumpkin soup, enchilada chicken soup

Replace Chinese takeaway with: Low-carb sweet and sour chicken

Replace rice with: Cauliflower rice

Replace mashed potatoes with: Cauliflower mashed potatoes

Replace burritos and tacos with: Flax tortillas, taco salad, psyllium husk tortillas

Replace bread and sandwiches with: Lettuce wraps, flax seed wraps, psyllium husk wraps

Replaces cookies with: Peanut butter cookies, low-carb cookies

Replace crackers with: Chia seed crackers, flaxseed crackers

Replace candy with: Mug cakes, fat bombs

Replace soda and fruit juice with: Smoothies, water, tea

Replace coffee with: Nothing, keep drinking it but just use Stevia as a sweetener!

Replace cocktails with: Dry wine, liquor

Replace ice cream with: Avocado ice cream, low-carb sorbet

Replace brownies with: Low-carb macadamia nut brownies, avocado brownies, almond flour brownies

Replace any pie crust with: Nut-based crusts

Replace custard with: Pots de Crème

Replace flour with: Almond flour

Replace breadcrumbs with: Pork rinds

Replace margarine and veg oil with: Butter, coconut oil

Replace sugar with: Stevia, erythritol

Replace chocolate with: Baker's chocolate, dark chocolate

Replace fruits with: Extracts

Replace cornstarch with: Xanthan gum

Replace high carb veg with: Dried spices

And there you have it, the complete cheat sheet for a ketogenic diet. It's a good idea to refer to this when you're not quite sure what to replace certain foods with – chances are it's on this list.

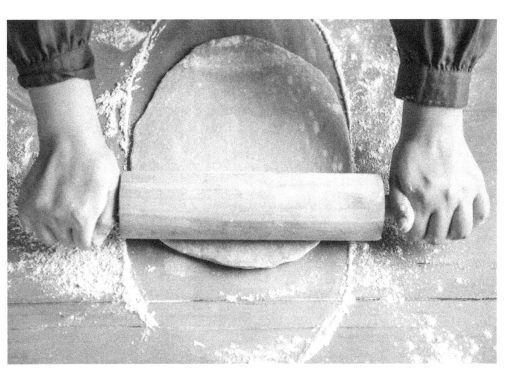

HOW TO REACH KETOSIS FASTER

Your goal with the ketogenic diet is to reach a state of ketosis. Here are a few tips on how to reach that state faster. Typically for your body to adjust and start up in a state of ketosis, it can take between 2 days and a week. However, the sooner, the better!

Carbs go down – The most important and most obvious way to reach ketosis faster is by making sure your carbs are going DOWN. You won't ever reach the state of ketosis while your carbs are high, so you must make sure you are heading toward 20grams a day. ALL the recipes in this book are lower than 10g.

Exercise – Becoming more active in your daily life can help you enter ketosis quicker. Alongside a lower carb intake, exercise helps your body increase its production of ketones which leads to entering a state of ketosis faster.

Up the fat – A lot of people fear fat, with the assumption that eating fat, makes you fat – it doesn't! Consuming more calories than you burn off, makes you fat. Getting healthy fats into your system will help you enter a state of ketosis quicker.

Mini fast – A lot of people have reported success on doing miniature fasts, where you simply cut your calories to around 1000 a day and use fats to make up most of that calorie count. This combo has helped a lot of people reach ketosis faster.

Stay hydrated and get your sleep – A lot of people will find that when cutting carbs that they soon become dehydrated. Dehydration can cause a whole host of issues and even affect your sleep which is vital for overall health – so make sure you get your water in.

Stop Worrying About Ketosis

To me, the ketogenic diet with all its rules and regulations sounds like a drag. Listening to Youtubers and 'experts' will have you believe that you can't take ANY enjoyment from your diet – and the only enjoyment you can have it those zero-sugar desserts that taste awful.

The problem with this is that when something becomes a chore, you'll more than likely give up on it. While there are some 'die-hard' keto people out there who can stick to the diet rigidly, it's not sustainable for your average Joe.

So, my proposal here is that you stop worrying about everything that goes in your mouth and enjoy the diet. Of course, eating an abundancy of high carb foods is eventually going to kick you out of ketosis, BUT, if this happens, don't worry – it will only take you around 3 days to enter a state of ketosis again. Plus, if you are already heavily into ketosis and have one high-carb meal, chances are you will remain in ketosis.

Try not to think of this as a 'diet' but more so a lifestyle change. Diets are short term and rarely ever last in the long run. If you can picture this as a marathon and not a sprint, you'll reap the amazing benefits on being in a state of ketosis.

With that brief thought in mind, let's get on with the recipes!

SIMPLE KETO BREAD

Preparation time: 10 minutes

Cooking time: 40 minutes

Servings: 6

Ingredients:

- ½ cup flaxseed meal
- 1 cup coconut flour
- 6 eggs, whisked
- ½ cup water
- 1 tablespoon apple cider vinegar
- 1 teaspoon baking powder
- 1 teaspoon baking soda
- A pinch of salt

Directions:

1. In a bowl, mix all the ingredients except the eggs and water and stir well.
2. Add the water gradually and stir well.
3. Also add the eggs and start kneading until you obtain a dough.
4. Transfer the dough to a round loaf pan and cook the bread at 350 degrees F for 40 minutes.
5. Cool the bread down, slice and serve it.

Nutrition: calories 423, fat 20, fiber 1, carbs 2, protein 30

FLAX SEED BREAD

Preparation time: 10 minutes

Cooking time: 20 minutes

Servings: 6

Ingredients:

- 2 cups flax seed, ground
- 1 tablespoon baking powder
- 1 and ½ cups protein isolate
- A pinch of salt
- 6 egg whites, whisked
- 1 egg, whisked
- ¾ cup water
- 3 tablespoons coconut oil, melted
- ¼ cup stevia

Directions:

1. In a bowl, mix all dry ingredients and stir well.
2. In a separate bowl, mix the egg whites and the rest of the wet ingredients, stir well and combine the 2 mixtures.
3. Stir the bread and mix well. Pour into a loaf pan and bake at 350 degrees F for 20 minutes.
4. Cool the bread down, slice and serve.

Nutrition: calories 263, fat 17, fiber 4, carbs 2, protein 20

DELICIOUS ROSEMARY FOCACCIA

Preparation time: 10 minutes

Cooking time: 25 minutes

Servings: 6

Ingredients:

- 1 cup flaxseed meal
- 1 cup almond flour
- ½ cup olive oil
- 2 garlic cloves, minced
- A pinch of salt and black pepper
- 1 and ½ tablespoons baking powder
- 6 eggs
- 1 teaspoon rosemary, chopped
- Cooking spray

Directions:

1. In a bowl, mix the flaxseed meal with almond flour, garlic, salt, pepper, baking powder and the rosemary and stir.
2. Add the eggs and stir everything.
3. Add the oil gradually at the end and whisk the batter really well.
4. Pour this into a square pan greased with cooking spray, spread well and bake at 350 degrees F for 25 minutes.
5. Slice and serve.

Nutrition: calories 243, fat 18, fiber 12, carbs 3, protein 10

LEMONY SHORTBREAD

Preparation time: 30 minutes

Cooking time: 15 minutes

Servings: 8

Ingredients:

- 6 tablespoons ghee, melted
- 2 cups almond flour
- 4 teaspoons lemon juice
- 1/3 cup stevia
- 1 tablespoon lemon zest, grated
- 1 teaspoon vanilla extract
- ½ teaspoon baking soda
- ½ teaspoon baking powder
- 2 teaspoons rosemary, dried

Directions:

1. In a bowl, mix the flour with lemon zest, vanilla extract, baking soda, baking powder and the rosemary and stir well.
2. Add the remaining ingredients, stir the dough well and shape a medium log out of this mix.
3. Wrap the log in plastic wrap and keep in the freezer for 30 minutes.
4. Unwrap the dough, cut into circles and arrange them on a lined baking sheet.
5. Bake at 360 degrees F for 15 minutes, cool the shortbread down and serve.

Nutrition: calories 130, fat 7, fiber 2, carbs 1, protein 3

FAST PUMPKIN BREAD

Preparation time: 10 minutes

Cooking time: 1 hour and 15 minutes

Servings: 8

Ingredients:

- 3 egg whites
- 1 and ½ cup almond flour
- ¼ cup pumpkin flesh
- ½ cup coconut milk
- ¼ cup swerve
- ¼ psyllium husk powder
- 2 teaspoons baking powder
- 1 and ½ teaspoons pumpkin pie spice
- A pinch of salt and white pepper

Directions:

1. In a bowl, mix the flour with swerve, psyllium husk powder, pumpkin pie spice, salt and pepper and stir well.
2. Add the rest of the ingredients and stir everything well.
3. Pour this into a lined loaf pan and bake at 350 degrees F for 1 hour and 15 minutes, cool down, slice and serve.

Nutrition: calories 115, fat 9, fiber 2, carbs 4, protein 5

ZUCCHINI BREAD

Preparation time: 10 minutes

Cooking time: 1 hour

Servings: 8

Ingredients:

- 3 cups almond flour
- 3 eggs
- ½ cup vegetable oil
- 1 and ½ cups erythritol
- A pinch of salt
- ½ teaspoon nutmeg, ground
- 1 and ½ teaspoons baking powder
- ¼ teaspoon ginger powder
- 1 teaspoon cinnamon powder
- ½ cup walnuts, chopped
- 1 cup zucchini, grated and pressed

Directions:

1. In a large bowl, mix the flour with erythritol, salt, nutmeg, baking powder, ginger and cinnamon powder and stir well.
2. Add the eggs, the oil gradually and the zucchinis and stir well.
3. Pour into a lined loaf pan, sprinkle the walnuts on top and cook at 350 degrees F for 1 hour.
4. Cool the bread down, slice and serve.

Nutrition: calories 200, fat 18, fiber 4, carbs 5, protein 7

Simple Keto Buns

Preparation time: 10 minutes

Cooking time: 12 minutes

Servings: 4

Ingredients:

- 2 eggs
- 2 tablespoons almond flour
- 2 tablespoons psyllium husk powder
- 2 tablespoons chicken stock
- ¼ teaspoon baking powder
- 2 tablespoons butter, melted

Directions:

1. In a bowl, mix all the ingredients and stir really well until you obtain a dough.
2. Divide the dough into 4 pieces and shape balls out of this mix.
3. Flatten the balls slightly, arrange them on a lined baking sheet and bake at 350 degrees f for 12 minutes.
4. Serve warm.

Nutrition: calories 243, fat 14, fiber 2, carbs 4, protein 8

BREAKFAST BAGELS

Preparation time: 10 minutes

Cooking time: 18 minutes

Servings: 4

Ingredients:

- 1 cup almond flour
- 1 egg
- 1 and ½ cups mozzarella, grated
- 2 tablespoons cream cheese
- 1 teaspoon stevia
- 1 tablespoon ghee, melted
- 1 tablespoon sesame seeds

Directions:

1. In a bowl, mix all the ingredients except the ghee and sesame seeds and stir well until you obtain a dough.
2. Divide the dough into 4 round pieces and arrange them in a donut pan.
3. Brush the bagels with the melted ghee, sprinkle the sesame seeds on top and bake at 390 degrees F for 18 minutes.
4. Serve for breakfast.

Nutrition: calories 245, fat 14, fiber 4, carbs 5, protein 14

ITALIAN BREADSTICKS

Preparation time: 10 minutes

Cooking time: 15 minutes

Servings: 6

Ingredients:

- 2 cups mozzarella cheese, grated
- 3 tablespoons cream cheese
- 1 cup almond flour
- 1 tablespoon psyllium husk powder
- 1 egg
- 1 teaspoon baking powder
- A pinch of salt and black pepper
- 2 tablespoons Italian seasoning

Directions:

1. In a bowl, mix the cheese with cream cheese, flour, psyllium husk powder, the egg, baking powder, salt, pepper and Italian seasoning and stir well.
2. Spread this on a lined baking sheet, press well and cut into medium pieces.
3. Cook the sticks at 400 degrees F for 15 minutes and serve cold.

Nutrition: calories 234, fat 12, fiber 3, carbs 4, protein 9

CHEESY BREADSTICKS

Preparation time: 10 minutes

Cooking time: 15 minutes

Servings: 6

Ingredients:

- 8 ounces mozzarella cheese, shredded
- 3 ounces cheddar cheese, shredded
- ¼ cup parmesan, grated
- 1 teaspoon garlic powder
- 1 cup coconut flour
- 3 tablespoons cream cheese
- 1 egg
- 1 teaspoon baking powder

Directions:

1. In a bowl, mix all the cheese and stir.
2. Add the rest of the ingredients and stir well.
3. Spread well into a lined square pan, press and cut into sticks.
4. Bake at 400 degrees F for 15 minutes and serve warm.

Nutrition: calories 314, fat 20, fiber 4, carbs 5, protein 16

BUTTERY BREADSTICKS

Preparation time: 10 minutes

Cooking time: 15 minutes

Servings: 6

Ingredients:

- 8 ounces cheddar cheese, shredded
- 2 tablespoons cinnamon powder
- 3 tablespoons butter, melted
- 6 tablespoons swerve
- 1 tablespoon psyllium husk powder
- 1 cup coconut flour
- 1 egg
- 3 tablespoons cream cheese
- 1 teaspoon baking powder

Directions:

1. In a bowl, mix the cheese with cinnamon, butter, swerve, husk powder, baking powder and coconut flour and stir well.
2. Add the egg and cream cheese and stir well.
3. Spread this into a lined baking sheet, press well, cut into sticks and bake at 390 degrees F for 15 minutes.
4. Serve warm.

Nutrition: calories 282, fat 18, fiber 3, carbs 4, protein 13

JALAPENO LOAF

Preparation time: 10 minutes

Cooking time: 22 minutes

Servings: 6

Ingredients:

- 1 and ½ cups almond flour
- ½ cup flaxseed meal
- A pinch of salt
- 2 teaspoons baking powder
- 4 tablespoons butter, melted
- ½ cup sour cream
- 4 eggs
- 10 drops stevia
- 2 jalapenos, chopped
- ½ cup cheddar, grated
- Cooking spray

Directions:

1. In a bowl, mix the flour with flaxseed meal, salt, baking powder, stevia, jalapenos and the cheese and stir.
2. Add the remaining ingredients and mix them until you obtain a dough.
3. Transfer it to a loaf pan greased with cooking spray and bake at 375 degrees F for 22 minutes.
4. Cool the bread down, slice and serve.

Nutrition: calories 300, fat 20, fiber 3, carbs 4, protein 12

FLUFFY KETO BREAD

Preparation time: 10 minutes

Cooking time: 1 hour and 5 minutes

Servings: 10

Ingredients:

- 1 and ¼ cups almond flour
- A pinch of salt
- 2 teaspoons apple cider vinegar
- 2 teaspoons baking powder
- 4 tablespoons psyllium husk powder
- 1 cup hot water
- 3 eggs, beaten well
- 2 tablespoons sesame seeds
- Cooking spray

Directions:

1. In a bowl, mix the flour with salt, baking powder, and husk powder and stir.
2. Add the rest of the ingredients except the sesame seeds and cooking spray and stir until you obtain a dough.
3. Transfer the dough to a loaf pan greased with cooking spray and bake at 350 degrees F for 1 hour and 5 minutes.
4. Cool the bread down, slice and serve.

Nutrition: calories 163, fat 4, fiber 4, carbs 6, protein 7

CHEESY BROCCOLI BREAD

Preparation time: 10 minutes

Cooking time: 15 minutes

Servings: 2

Ingredients:

- Cooking spray
- 1 egg
- 1 tablespoon coconut flour
- 1 tablespoon almond flour
- 1 tablespoon almond milk
- 1 tablespoon butter, melted
- ¼ teaspoon baking powder
- A pinch of salt
- 1 tablespoon broccoli, chopped
- 1 tablespoon mozzarella, grated

Directions:

1. In a bowl mix the coconut flour with the almond flour, baking powder, salt, broccoli and the mozzarella and stir.
2. Add the remaining ingredients except the cooking spray and stir everything really well.
3. Grease a loaf pan with cooking spray, pour the bread batter, cook at 400 degrees F for 15 minutes, cool down and serve.

Nutrition: calories 244, fat 20, fiber 4, carbs 6, protein 6

COCONUT BREAD

Preparation time: 10 minutes

Cooking time: 45 minutes

Servings: 6

Ingredients:

- 1 cup coconut flour
- 8 tablespoons ghee, melted
- 6 eggs
- 2 teaspoons oregano, dried
- 1 teaspoon baking powder
- 1 teaspoon garlic powder
- A pinch of salt

Directions:

1. In a bowl, mix the flour with oregano, baking powder, garlic powder and the salt and stir.
2. Add the eggs and ghee, stir until you obtain a dough, and transfer to a lined loaf pan.
3. Cook at 350 degrees F for 45 minutes, cool down, slice and serve.

Nutrition: calories 183, fat 12, fiber 2, carbs 4, protein 6

DUTCH OVEN BREAD

Preparation time: 20 minutes

Cooking time: 30 minutes

Servings: 6

Ingredients:

- 1 teaspoon baking powder
- 1 teaspoon baking soda
- 3 cups almond flour
- 1 and ½ cups warm water
- A pinch of salt
- 1 teaspoon stevia

Directions:

1. In a bowl, mix the water with the flour and stir well.
2. Add the rest of the ingredients, stir until you obtain a dough and leave aside for 20 minutes.
3. Transfer the dough to a Dutch oven and bake the bread at 400 degrees F for 30 minutes.
4. Cool the bread down, slice and serve.

Nutrition: calories 143, fat 9, fiber 3, carbs 4, protein 6

Simple Avocado Bread

Preparation time: 10 minutes

Cooking time: 40 minutes

Servings: 6

Ingredients:

- 1 cup coconut flour
- ½ teaspoon baking soda
- ½ teaspoon baking powder
- ¼ teaspoon cinnamon powder
- ¼ cup ghee, melted
- ½ cup swerve
- 1 egg
- ¼ teaspoon vanilla extract
- 1 cup avocado, peeled, pitted and mashed
- 1 teaspoon lime juice

Directions:

1. In a bowl, mix the flour with baking powder, baking soda, cinnamon and vanilla extract and stir well.
2. Add the remaining ingredients and mix the dough really well.
3. Transfer the dough to a lined loaf pan and bake at 325 degrees F for 40 minutes.
4. Cool the bread down, slice and serve.

Nutrition: calories 235, fat 12, fiber 3, carbs 5, protein 5

ARTICHOKE BREAD

Preparation time: 10 minutes

Cooking time: 30 minutes

Servings: 10

Ingredients:

- 14 ounces canned artichoke hearts, drained and chopped
- 1 garlic clove, minced
- 1 cup parmesan, grated
- 1 cup almond flour
- ½ teaspoon baking powder
- 1 and ½ cups warm water

Directions:

1. In a bowl, mix the flour with baking powder, and the water and stir well.
2. Add the rest of the ingredients, stir the dough well and transfer it to a lined round pan.
3. Bake at 360 degrees F for 30 minutes, cool the bread down, slice and serve.

Nutrition: calories 211, fat 12, fiber 3, carbs 5, protein 6

CAULIFLOWER BREAD

Preparation time: 10 minutes

Cooking time: 50 minutes

Servings: 4

Ingredients:

- 6 eggs, whisked
- 6 tablespoons olive oil
- 3 cups cauliflower, riced
- 1 and ¼ cup almond flour
- A pinch of salt
- 1 tablespoon baking powder

Directions:

1. In a large bowl, mix the flour with salt, baking powder and cauliflower rice and stir well.
2. Add the rest of the ingredients, stir well and pour the batter in a lined loaf pan.
3. Cook the bread at 350 degrees F for 50 minutes, cool down, slice and serve.

Nutrition: calories 204, fat 14, fiber 2 carbs 6, protein 7

VEGGIE BREAD

Preparation time: 10 minutes

Cooking time: 30 minutes

Servings: 12

Ingredients:

- ½ teaspoon baking powder
- ½ teaspoon baking soda
- 5 ounces almond milk
- 1/3 cup water, warm
- ¼ cup coconut oil, melted
- 1 cup cabbage, shredded
- 1 egg, whisked
- 4 cups almond flour
- 1 tablespoon stevia
- ¼ cup parsley, chopped

Directions:

1. In a large bowl, mix the baking powder with baking soda, flour, and stevia and stir.
2. Add the milk and water and start kneading the dough.
3. Add the rest of the ingredients, knead the dough well and transfer it to a lined loaf pan.
4. Cook at 350 degrees F for 30 minutes, cool the bread down, slice and serve it.

Nutrition: calories 138, fat 5, fiber 2, carbs 6, protein 7

Cheesy Broccoli Bread 2

Preparation time: 10 minutes

Cooking time: 30 minutes

Servings: 4

Ingredients:

- 5 eggs, whisked
- 2 teaspoons baking powder
- 1 cup cheddar, shredded
- 1 cup broccoli florets, separated
- 4 tablespoons coconut flour
- Cooking spray

Directions:

1. In a bowl, mix all the ingredients except the cooking spray and stir really well.
2. Pour the batter in a loaf pan greased with cooking spray and bake at 350 degrees F for 30 minutes.
3. Cool the bread down, slice and serve.

Nutrition: calories 123, fat 6, fiber 1, carbs 3, protein 6

KETO SPINACH BREAD

Preparation time: 10 minutes

Cooking time: 30 minutes

Servings: 10

Ingredients:

- ½ cup spinach, chopped
- 1 tablespoon olive oil
- 1 cup water
- 3 cups almond flour
- A pinch of salt and black pepper
- 1 tablespoon stevia
- 1 teaspoon baking powder
- 1 teaspoon baking soda
- ½ cup cheddar, shredded

Directions:

1. In a bowl, mix the flour, with salt, pepper, stevia, baking powder, baking soda and the cheddar and stir well.
2. Add the remaining ingredients, stir the batter really well and pour it into a lined loaf pan.
3. Cook at 350 degrees F for 30 minutes, cool the bread down, slice and serve.

Nutrition: calories 142, fat 7, fiber 3, carbs 5, protein 6

CINNAMON ASPARAGUS BREAD

Preparation time: 10 minutes

Cooking time: 45 minutes

Servings: 8

Ingredients:

- 1 cup stevia
- ¾ cup coconut oil, melted
- 1 and ½ cups almond flour
- 2 eggs, whisked
- A pinch of salt
- 1 teaspoon baking soda
- 1 teaspoon cinnamon powder
- 2 cups asparagus, chopped
- Cooking spray

Directions:

1. In a bowl, mix all the ingredients except the cooking spray and stir the batter really well.
2. Pour this batter into a loaf pan greased with cooking spray and bake at 350 degrees F for 45 minutes, cool the bread down, slice and serve.

Nutrition: calories 165, fat 6, fiber 3, carbs 5, protein 6

KALE AND CHEESE BREAD

Preparation time: 10 minutes

Cooking time: 1 hour

Servings: 8

Ingredients:

- 2 cups kale, chopped
- 1 cup warm water
- 1 teaspoon baking powder
- 1 teaspoon baking soda
- 2 tablespoons olive oil
- 2 teaspoons stevia
- 1 cup parmesan, grated
- 3 cups almond flour
- A pinch of salt
- 1 egg
- 2 tablespoons basil, chopped

Directions:

1. In a bowl, mix the flour, salt, parmesan, stevia, baking soda and baking powder and stir.
2. Add the rest of the ingredients gradually and stir the dough well.
3. Transfer it to a lined loaf pan, cook at 350 degrees F for 1 hour, cool down, slice and serve.

Nutrition: calories 231, fat 7, fiber 2, carbs 5, protein 7

BEET BREAD

Preparation time: 1 hour and 10 minutes

Cooking time: 35 minutes

Servings: 6

Ingredients:

- 1 cup warm water
- 3 and ½ cups almond flour
- 1 and ½ cups beet puree
- 2 tablespoons olive oil
- A pinch of salt
- 1 teaspoon stevia
- 1 teaspoon baking powder
- 1 teaspoon baking soda

Directions:

1. In a bowl, mix the flour with the water and beet puree and stir well.
2. Add the rest of the ingredients, stir the dough well and pour it into a lined loaf pan.
3. Leave the mix to rise in a warm place for 1 hour, and then bake the bread at 375 degrees F for 35 minutes.
4. Cool the bread down, slice and serve.

Nutrition: calories 200, fat 8, fiber 3, carbs 5, protein 6

KETO CELERY BREAD

Preparation time: 2 hours and 10 minutes

Cooking time: 35 minutes

Servings: 6

Ingredients:

- ½ cup celery, chopped
- 3 cups almond flour
- 1 teaspoon baking powder
- 1 teaspoon baking soda
- A pinch of salt
- 2 tablespoons coconut oil, melted
- ½ cup celery puree

Directions:

1. In a bowl, mix the flour with salt, baking powder and baking soda and stir.
2. Add the rest of the ingredients, stir the dough well, cover the bowl and keep in a warm place for 2 hours.
3. Transfer the dough to a lined loaf pan and cook at 400 degrees F for 35 minutes.
4. Cool the bread down, slice and serve.

Nutrition: calories 162, fat 6, fiber 2, carbs 6, protein 4

Easy Cucumber Bread

Preparation time: 10 minutes

Cooking time: 50 minutes

Servings: 6

Ingredients:

- 1 cup erythritol
- 1 cup coconut oil, melted
- 1 cup almonds, chopped
- 1 teaspoon vanilla extract
- A pinch of salt
- A pinch of nutmeg, ground
- ½ teaspoon baking powder
- A pinch of cloves
- 3 eggs
- 1 teaspoon baking soda
- 1 tablespoon cinnamon powder
- 2 cups cucumber, peeled, deseeded and shredded
- 3 cups coconut flour
- Cooking spray

Directions:

1. In a bowl, mix the flour with cucumber, cinnamon, baking soda, cloves, baking powder, nutmeg, salt, vanilla extract and the almonds and stir well.
2. Add the rest of the ingredients except the coconut flour, stir well and transfer the dough to a loaf pan greased with cooking spray.

3. Bake at 325 degrees F for 50 minutes, cool the bread down, slice and serve.

Nutrition: calories 243, fat 12, fiber 3, carbs 6, protein 7

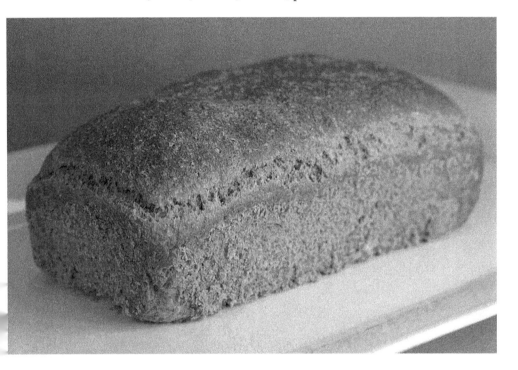

RED BELL PEPPER BREAD

Preparation time: 10 minutes

Cooking time: 30 minutes

Servings: 12

Ingredients:

- 1 and ½ cups red bell peppers, chopped
- 1 teaspoon baking powder
- 1 teaspoon baking soda
- 2 tablespoons warm water
- 1 and ¼ cups parmesan, grated
- A pinch of salt
- 4 cups almond flour
- 2 tablespoons ghee, melted
- 1/3 cup almond milk
- 1 egg

Directions:

1. In a bowl, mix the flour with salt, parmesan, baking powder, baking soda and the bell peppers and stir well.
2. Add the rest of the ingredients and stir the bread batter well.
3. Transfer it to a lined loaf pan and bake at 350 degrees F for 30 minutes.
4. Cool the bread down, slice and serve.

Nutrition: calories 100, fat 5, fiber 1, carbs 4, protein 4

Tomato Bread

Preparation time: 1 hour and 10 minutes

Cooking time: 35 minutes

Servings: 12

Ingredients:

- 6 cups almond flour
- ½ teaspoon basil, dried
- ¼ teaspoon rosemary, dried
- 1 teaspoon oregano, dried
- ½ teaspoon garlic powder
- 2 tablespoons olive oil
- 2 cups tomato juice
- ½ cup tomato sauce
- 1 teaspoon baking powder
- 1 teaspoon baking soda
- 3 tablespoons swerve

Directions:

1. In a bowl, mix the flour with basil, rosemary, oregano and garlic and stir.
2. Add the rest of the ingredients and stir the batter well.
3. Pour into a lined loaf pan, cover and keep in a warm place for 1 hour.
4. Bake the bread at 375 degrees F for 35 minutes, cool down, slice and serve.

Nutrition: calories 102, fat 5, fiber 3, carbs 7, protein 4

HERBED KETO BREAD

Preparation time: 1 hour and 30 minutes

Cooking time: 40 minutes

Servings: 8

Ingredients:

- 3 cups coconut flour
- 1 teaspoon baking powder
- 1 teaspoon baking soda
- 2 teaspoons stevia
- 1 and ½ cups warm water
- ½ teaspoon basil, dried
- 1 teaspoon oregano, dried
- ½ teaspoon thyme, dried
- ½ teaspoon marjoram, dried
- 2 tablespoons olive oil

Directions:

1. In a bowl, mix the flour with baking powder, baking soda, stevia, basil oregano, thyme, and the marjoram and stir.
2. Add the remaining ingredients, mix the dough, cover and keep in a warm place for 1 hour and 30 minutes.
3. Transfer the dough to a floured working surface and knead it again for 2-3 minutes.
4. Transfer to a lined loaf pan and bake at 400 degrees F for 40 minutes.
5. Cool the bread down before serving.

Nutrition: calories 200, fat 7, fiber 3, carbs 5, protein 6

OLIVE BREAD

Preparation time: 10 minutes

Cooking time: 45 minutes

Servings: 12

Ingredients:

- 1 teaspoon baking powder
- 1 and ½ cups warm water
- A pinch of salt
- 3 cups almond flour
- 1 cup black olives, pitted and sliced

Directions:

1. In a large bowl, mix all the ingredients and knead until you obtain a dough.
2. Cover the bowl, keep the dough in a warm place for 40 minutes and then transfer it to a lined round loaf pan.
3. Bake the bread at 400 degrees F for 40 minutes, cool it down, slice and serve.

Nutrition: calories 222, fat 7, fiber 3, carbs 5, protein 6

GREEN OLIVE BREAD

Preparation time: 10 minutes

Cooking time: 45 minutes

Servings: 10

Ingredients:

- 3 cups almond flour
- A pinch of salt
- ½ teaspoon baking powder
- 1 and ½ cups warm water
- 3 tablespoons rosemary, chopped
- ½ cup green olives, pitted and chopped
- A pinch of salt and black pepper

Directions:

1. In a bowl, mix the flour with salt, rosemary and baking powder and stir.
2. Add the rest of the ingredients, mix the dough well and transfer it to a lined loaf pan.
3. Bake at 400 degrees F for 45 minutes, cool down, slice and serve.

Nutrition: calories 204, fat 12, fiber 4, carbs 5, protein 7

DELICIOUS EGGPLANT BREAD

Preparation time: 10 minutes

Cooking time: 1 hour

Servings: 12

Ingredients:

- 4 eggs, whisked
- 1 cup erythritol
- ½ cup ghee, melted
- ½ cup coconut oil, melted
- 2 cups eggplant, peeled and grated
- 1 tablespoon vanilla extract
- 2 cups almond flour
- 1 and ½ teaspoon cinnamon powder
- ¼ teaspoon nutmeg, ground
- ½ teaspoon baking powder
- 1 teaspoon baking soda
- A pinch of salt
- ½ cup pine nuts
- Cooking spray

Directions:

1. In a bowl, mix the flour with cinnamon, nutmeg, baking powder, baking soda, salt, pine nuts and the vanilla and stir.
2. Add the rest of the ingredients except the cooking spray, mix the batter well and pour into a loaf pan greased with the cooking spray.
3. Cook at 350 degrees F for 1 hour, cool down, slice and serve.

Nutrition: calories 200, fat 7, fiber 3, carbs 5, protein 6

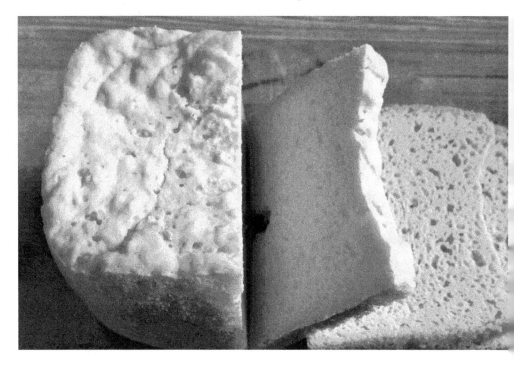

GREAT BLACKBERRIES BREAD

Preparation time: 10 minutes

Cooking time: 1 hour

Servings: 10

Ingredients:

- 2 cups almond flour
- ½ cup stevia
- 1 and ½ teaspoons baking powder
- 1 teaspoon baking soda
- 2 eggs, whisked
- 1 and ½ cups almond flour
- ¼ cup ghee, melted
- 1 tablespoon vanilla extract
- 1 cup blackberries, mashed
- Cooking spray

Directions:

1. In a bowl, mix the flour with the baking powder, baking soda, stevia, vanilla and blackberries and stir well.
2. Add the rest of the ingredients, stir the batter and pour it into a loaf pan greased with cooking spray.
3. Bake at 400 degrees F for 1 hour, cool down, slice and serve.

Nutrition: calories 200, fat 7, fiber 3, carbs 5, protein 7

KETO RASPBERRIES BREAD

Preparation time: 10 minutes

Cooking time: 50 minutes

Servings: 6

Ingredients:

- 2 cups almond flour
- 1 teaspoon baking soda
- ¾ cup erythritol
- A pinch of salt
- 1 egg
- ¾ cup coconut milk
- ¼ cup ghee, melted
- 2 cups raspberries
- 2 teaspoons vanilla extract
- ¼ cup coconut oil, melted

Directions:

1. In a bowl, mix the flour with the baking soda, erythritol, salt, vanilla and the raspberries and stir.
2. Add the rest of the ingredients gradually and mix the batter well.
3. Pour this into a lined loaf pan and bake at 350 degrees F for 50 minutes.
4. Cool the bread down, slice and serve.

Nutrition: calories 200, fat 7, fiber 3, carbs 5, protein 7

SIMPLE STRAWBERRY BREAD

Preparation time: 10 minutes

Cooking time: 50 minutes

Servings: 8

Ingredients:

- 3 and ½ cups almond flour
- 2 cups strawberries, chopped
- 1 teaspoon baking soda
- 2 cups swerve
- 1 tablespoon cinnamon powder
- 4 eggs, whisked
- 1 and ¼ cups coconut oil, melted
- Cooking spray

Directions:

1. In a bowl, mix the flour with baking soda, swerve, strawberries and the cinnamon and stir.
2. Add the remaining ingredients, stir the batter and pour this into 2 loaf pans greased with cooking spray.
3. Bake at 350 degrees F for 50 minutes, cool the bread down, slice and serve.

Nutrition: calories 221, fat 7, fiber 4, carbs 5, protein 3

GREAT PLUM BREAD

Preparation time: 10 minutes

Cooking time: 50 minutes

Servings: 8

Ingredients:

- 1 cup plums, pitted and chopped
- 1 and ½ cups coconut flour
- ¼ teaspoon baking soda
- ½ cup ghee, melted
- A pinch of salt
- 1 and ¼ cups swerve
- ½ teaspoon vanilla extract
- 1/3 cup coconut cream
- 2 eggs, whisked

Directions:

1. In a bowl, mix the flour with baking soda, salt, swerve, and the vanilla and stir.
2. In a separate bowl, mix the plums with the remaining ingredients and stir.
3. Combine the 2 mixtures and stir the batter well.
4. Pour into 2 lined loaf pans and bake at 350 degrees F for 50 minutes.
5. Cool the bread down, slice and serve them.

Nutrition: calories 199, fat 8, fiber 3, carbs 6, protein 4

LIME BREAD

Preparation time: 10 minutes

Cooking time: 50 minutes

Servings: 8

Ingredients:

- 2/3 cup ghee, melted
- 2 cups swerve
- 4 eggs, whisked
- 3 teaspoons baking powder
- 1 cup almond milk
- 2 tablespoons lime zest, grated
- 2 tablespoons lime juice
- 3 cups coconut flour
- Cooking spray

Directions:

1. In a bowl, mix the flour with lime zest, baking powder and the swerve and stir.
2. In a separate bowl, mix the lime juice with the rest of the ingredients except the cooking spray and stir well.
3. Combine the 2 mixtures, stir the batter well and pour into 2 loaf pans greased with cooking spray and bake at 350 degrees F for 50 minutes.
4. Cool the bread down, slice and serve.

Nutrition: calories 203, fat 7, fiber 3, carbs 4, protein 6

DELICIOUS RHUBARB BREAD

Preparation time: 10 minutes

Cooking time: 40 minutes

Servings: 10

Ingredients:

- 1 cup almond milk
- 1 teaspoon vanilla extract
- 1 tablespoon lemon juice
- 2/3 cup coconut oil, melted
- 1 egg
- 1 and ½ cups swerve
- 2 an ½ cups coconut flour
- A pinch of salt
- 2 cups rhubarb, chopped
- 1 teaspoon baking soda
- ½ teaspoon cinnamon powder
- 1 tablespoon ghee, melted
- Cooking spray

Directions:

1. In a bowl, mix the vanilla with lemon juice, swerve, flour, salt, rhubarb, baking soda, and the cinnamon and stir.
2. Add the rest of the ingredients except the cooking spray, stir the batter and pour into a loaf pan greased with cooking spray.
3. Bake at 350 degrees F for 40 minutes, cool down, slice and serve.

Nutrition: calories 200, fat 7, fiber 2, carbs 4, protein 6

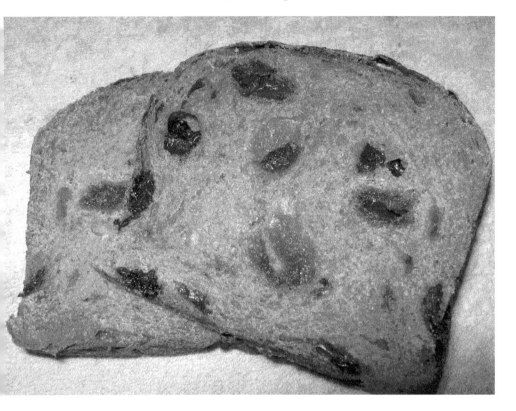

DELICIOUS CANTALOUPE BREAD

Preparation time: 10 minutes

Cooking time: 1 hour

Servings: 8

Ingredients:

- 4 tablespoons stevia
- 3 eggs
- 1 cup coconut oil, melted
- 1 tablespoon vanilla extract
- 1 teaspoon baking powder
- 1 teaspoon baking soda
- 2 teaspoons cinnamon powder
- ½ teaspoon ginger, ground
- 2 cups cantaloupe, peeled and pureed
- ½ cup ghee, melted
- 3 cups almond flour

Directions:

1. In a bowl, mix the flour with ginger, cinnamon, baking soda, baking powder, vanilla and the stevia and stir.
2. Add the rest of the ingredients and stir the batter well.
3. Pour into 2 lined loaf pans and bake at 360 degrees F for 1 hour.
4. Cool the bread down, slice and serve.

Nutrition: calories 211, fat 8, fiber 3, carbs 6, protein 6

Thanks everyone!

Making bread can be so much fun! You can use so many different ingredients and flavors! The combinations are endless! The bread recipes collection you've just discovered shows you how to make the most delicious and textured ketogenic breads from the comfort of your own kitchen.

Anyone can enjoy these breads and you don't need to be an expert in the kitchen to make them. The Ketogenic breads gathered here are all so rich and delightful! Check out all of them and enjoy them!

Please continue reading for an awesome bonus…

FREE FAT BOMB RECIPES BONUS!

CHOCOLATE PEPPERMINT BOMBS

Ingredients (serves 19)

Filling:

½ cup coconut oil
½ cup coconut butter
12 drops Stevia
1 tsp peppermint extract

Coating:

½ cup coconut oil
½ cup cacao powder
20 drops Stevia
1 tsp vanilla extract

Instructions

1. Melt the coconut oil and coconut butter together in a saucepan over a medium heat.

2. Transfer to a mixing bowl and add in the Stevia and peppermint extract. Mix well.

3. Spoon mixture into an ice cube tray or small cupcake liners. Use 2 tablespoons per mold. Freeze for 1 hour.

4. Meanwhile, mix together all the COATING ingredients in a mixing bowl. You will need to melt the coconut oil first.

5. Remove the now firm filling mixture from their mold and dip each one into the coating mixture. You can use a fork for this. Place on parchment paper and freeze when all are covered.

6. Serve when coating is solid!

Calories: 130 Carbs: 2g Fiber: 1g Fat: 13g Saturated Fat: 10g

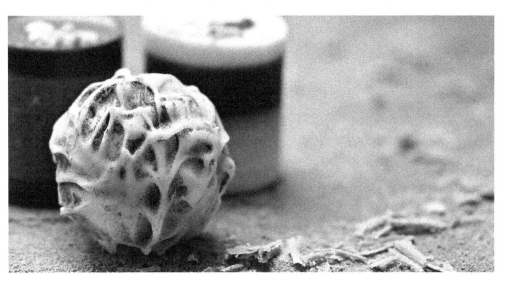

3 INGREDIENTS ONLY BOMBS

Ingredients (serves 12)

1 cup almond butter
½ cup coconut flour
2 tablespoons Stevia

Instructions

1. Line a baking sheet with parchment paper.

2. Whisk together the butter, Stevia and coconut flour in a small bowl. Mix until thick, then allow to freeze for 15 minutes.

3. When 15 minutes is up, remove from freezer and roll into 12 small balls with your hands.

4. Place each ball onto the baking sheet then place back in freezer for 20 minutes until firm, then serve!

Calories: 75 Carbs: 1g Fat: 9g Saturated Fat: 4g Protein: 1.5g

MOCHA BOMBS

Ingredients (serves 12)

1 cup cream cheese
4 tablespoons Swerve
2 tablespoons unsweetened cocoa
¼ cup coffee, chilled
½ cup dark chocolate, melted
1/8 cup cocoa butter, melted

Instructions

1. In a blender, mix together the coffee, cream cheese, cocoa and Swerve. Blend until smooth.

2. Roll out 12 small fat bombs from the mixture onto a plate lined with parchment paper.

3. Now mix together the melted dark chocolate and cocoa butter.

4. Roll each ball through the mixture in step 3 until fully covered. Place back on plate when all 12 are done.

5. Allow to set in freezer for 2 hours. Serve when ready!

Calories: 105 Carbs: 2.3g Fat: 12g Protein: 2g Fiber: 0.7g

PUMPKIN CHEESECAKE BOMBS

Ingredients (serves 14)

8 ounces cream cheese
4 tablespoons Swerve
1/3 cup pumpkin puree
1 tsp pumpkin pie spice
1 tsp vanilla extract
2.5 tablespoons coconut flour
1/3 cup pecans, minced
1 tsp cinnamon
2 tablespoons Erythritol

Instructions

1. Line a baking sheet with parchment paper

2. With an electric mixer, beat together the cream cheese, swerve, pumpkin puree, pie spice, vanilla extract and coconut flour.

3. Place mixture and bowl in freezer for 15 minutes until the mixture is semi-firm. Meanwhile, combine the pecans, cinnamon and Erythritol in a separate bowl.

4. Remove mixture from freezer and form 14 small balls from it with your hands. Now roll each one into the pecan, cinnamon and Erythritol mixture until fully covered.

5. Re-freeze for 20 minutes then serve when desired!

Calories: 80 Carbs: 1.4g Fat: 9g Protein: 1.5g Fiber: 0.5g

Salted Caramel Peanut Butter bombs

Ingredients (serves 18)

8 tablespoons butter, unsalted
1 cup coconut oil
1 cup natural chunky peanut butter
¼ cup sugar-free caramel syrup

Instructions

1. Over a medium heat, melt all the ingredients into a saucepan and mix thoroughly.

2. Pour mixture into ice-cube tray and place in the freezer for 1 hour or until visibly set.

3. Remove when firm and serve when desired!

Calories: 125 Carbs: 2.3g Fat: 22g Protein: 3g Fiber: 0.7g

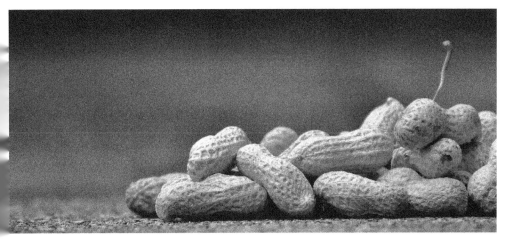

Chocolate Coconut Almond Bombs

Ingredients (serves 30)

½ cup coconut butter, melted
½ cup coconut oil, melted
1 tsp almond extract
¼ cup cocoa powder, unsweetened
½ tsp vanilla extract
10 drops Stevia
¼ cup almonds, crushed
¼ cup shredded coconut, unsweetened
¼ cup cacao nibs

Instructions

1. Melt the coconut butter and coconut oil over a medium heat in a saucepan. Then transfer it to a mixing bowl along with the cocoa powder, almond extract, vanilla extract and Stevia. Mix thoroughly.

2. Add the remaining ingredients and combine.

3. Fill mini cupcake liners with 1 tablespoon of mixture for each. This recipe should make around 30.

4. Leave to firm in freezer for 30 minutes before serving.

Calories: 87 Carbs: 1g Fat: 7g Protein: 0.3g Fiber: 1g

BLACKBERRY FAT BOMBS

Ingredients (serves 16)

1 cup coconut butter
1 cup coconut oil
½ tsp Stevia drops
½ cup frozen blackberries
½ tsp vanilla extract
1 tablespoon lemon juice

Instructions

1. Heat the coconut oil, coconut butter and frozen berries in a saucepan over a medium heat and stir until well combined.

2. Transfer the above mixture to a blender and add the remaining ingredients. Blend until smooth.

3. Pour the mixture out evenly into a pan lined with parchment paper. A 6x6 pan should be fine here.

4. Refrigerate for 1 hour. Remove when hardened and cut into 16 squares before serving!

Calories: 150 Carbs: 2.8g Fat: 17g Protein: 1g

Sea Salted Chocolate Bombs

Ingredients (serves 10)

½ cup whipping cream
½ cup coconut oil
½ cup sunflower butter
1 tsp vanilla extract
2 tablespoons cocoa powder
1/3 cup cream cheese
1 tsp cinnamon
3 tablespoons grass-fed butter
2 tsp coarse sea salt

Instructions

1. In a medium sized bowl, whip the whipping cream until peaks form. Fold in the vanilla extract.

2. In a blender, mix together the remaining ingredients MINUS the sea salt. Blend until smooth.

3. Fold this mixture slowly into the whipping cream in step 1 and combine thoroughly.

4. Spoon mixture into silicone molds. This recipe should make around 10 fat bombs.

5. Sprinkle each with some sea salt then freeze for 6-8 hours before serving!

Calories: 102 Carbs: 2.8g Fat: 19g Protein: 1g

Vanilla Cheesecake Bombs

Ingredients (serves 16)

8 ounces cream cheese
½ cup Splenda
1 cup heavy cream
2 tsp vanilla extract

Instructions

1. Add the cream cheese, Splenda and vanilla extract to a bowl and mix with a hand blender until smooth.

2. Add in the heavy cream and whisk until mixture is thick and produces firm peaks.

3. Spoon mixture into mini cupcake liners. If you can use a piping bag, then that's even better. This recipe should make around 16-20 fat bombs.

4. Set in fridge for 2 hours before serving!

Calories: 80 Carbs: 1g Fat: 10g Protein: 1g

SMOOTH AND CRUNCHY PECAN FAT BOMBS

Ingredients (serves 12)

½ cup pecans
¼ cup ghee
¼ cup coconut butter
1/8 tsp salt
¼ cup coconut oil
½ tsp vanilla extract

Instructions

1. Toast the pecans in a skillet over a medium heat until darker. They should smell toasty when ready.

2. Now chop the pecans into reasonably large chunks. This comes down to personal preference, how big you have them.

3. In a different saucepan, melt the coconut butter, ghee and coconut oil together over a low heat. Now stir in the vanilla and salt.

4. Divide out the chopped pecans into the silicon mold of your choice. I prefer using a cubed mold that holds 12 for this recipe.

5. Pour the mixture over the pecans evenly then leave to freeze for 30 minutes until hard.

6. If you don't have a mold, you can simply freeze the mixture in a container then chop it up afterwards!

Calories: 142 Carbs: 2g Fat: 16g Saturated fat: 10g Fiber: 1g Protein: 1g

KEY LIME PIE BOMBS

Ingredients (serves 30)

2 cups raw cashews
½ cup coconut butter
1 cup coconut oil
¾ cup key lime juice
¼ tsp Stevia

Instructions

1. Boil the cashew nuts for 12 minutes.

2. Melt the coconut oil over a medium heat in a saucepan.

3. Transfer the melted coconut oil to a food processor with all other ingredients, including cashews and blend until smooth.

4. Transfer mixture to a mixing bowl and leave in freezer for 30 minutes.

5. Form as many small balls as you can from the mixture. This recipe should make about 30 small fat bombs. Return these to the freezer for 20 minutes so they harden.

6. When ready to serve, leave them out to thaw a little beforehand.

Calories: 152 Carbs: 4g Fat: 15g Protein: 2g

Keto Mousse Bomb

Ingredients (serves 2)

1 cup full fat mascarpone cheese
1 tablespoon Erythritol
1 tsp baking cocoa powder

Instructions

1. Simply mix together the mascarpone cheese, cocoa powder and Erythritol until mixture is smooth.

2. Leave in fridge for 10 mins before consuming!

Calories: 252 Carbs: 2g Fat: 25g Protein: 1.5g Fiber: 3.4g

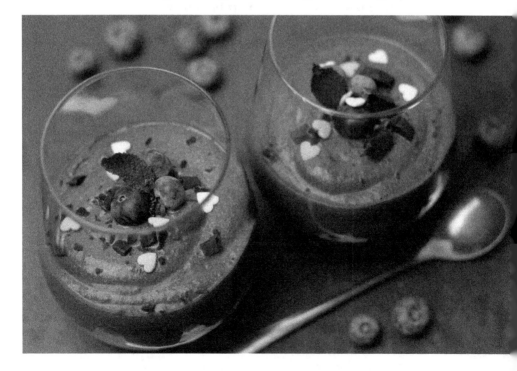

Pumpkin Pie Fat Bombs

Ingredients (serves 12)

½ cup shredded coconut, unsweetened
½ cup coconut oil
¼ cup collagen
20 drops Stevia
¼ tsp Himalayan salt
¾ cup pumpkin puree
1 tablespoon ground cinnamon
1 tsp ground ginger
¼ tsp vanilla extract
Pinch of ground cloves

Instructions

1. Line baking sheet with 12 mini muffin silicon molds.

2. In a blender, mix together the coconut oil, Stevia, shredded coconut and salt until smooth and drippy.

3. Remove a quarter cup of the above mixture, then add the remaining ingredients and blend again.

4. Pour this mixture evenly into the 12 molds. Press the mixture firmly into the mold.

5. Now, with the remaining quarter cup from step 3, pour this over the top of each fat bomb. This will create a layered effect.

6. Place on baking sheet then leave in freezer for 1 hour, then serve!

Calories: 202 Carbs: 2g Fat: 21g Protein: 3.5g Fiber: 3.4g

PECAN PEANUT CRUNCH FAT BOMBS

Ingredients (serves 16)

2 cups chopped pecan nuts
4 tablespoons melted coconut oil
2 tablespoons melted grass-fed butter
2 tablespoon peanut butter (sugar-free if possible)
2 tablespoon cocoa powder, unsweetened
½ tsp Stevia powder

Instructions

1. Melt the coconut oil and butter in a saucepan over medium heat, stirring well.

2. Finely chop the pecan nuts, then mix ALL the ingredients together in a medium-sized mixing bowl until fully combined.

3. Spoon the mixture into small cupcake molds, about 1 tablespoon per mold made me 16 fat bombs.

4. Leave in freezer for 15 minutes until firm.

5. Serve when desired. These can be stored in fridge or freezer.

Calories: 130 Carbs: 2.4g Fat: 15g Protein: 1.5g

COFFEE CHEESECAKE FAT BOMBS

Ingredients (serves 17)

2 cups cream cheese
1 cup grass-fed butter
1/3 cup Stevia
2 tablespoons cocoa powder, unsweetened
3 tablespoons cold brew coffee

Instructions

1. Mix together the cream cheese, grass-fed butter and Stevia in a medium-sized bowl. Use a blender for best results.

2. Scoop out one cup of the above mixture and transfer it to a small bowl. Now add the cocoa powder to this mixture and stir until combined.

3. Add the cold coffee brew to the medium-sized bowl in step 1 and stir until combined.

4. For the best results, use a casserole dish of an 8"x8" size and line it with parchment paper.

5. Line the bottom of the casserole dish with the cocoa mixture from step 2. This is your base, so to speak.

6. Now spread the other mixture over the top of this base, covering entirely.

7. Leave in freezer for 4 hours. Cut into squares when ready then serve.

Calories: 180 Carbs: 1.4g Fat: 20g Saturated Fat: 12g Protein: 1.5g

FERRERO ROCHER FAT BOMBS

Ingredients (serves 10)

¾ cup ground hazelnuts
3 tablespoons coconut oil
2 tablespoons Erythritol
1 ounce dark chocolate (85% cocoa)
½ tsp vanilla extract
½ tablespoon baking cocoa powder
½ cup chopped whole nuts and hazelnuts

Instructions

1. Melt the dark chocolate and coconut oil in a microwave or saucepan until fully melted.

2. Blend together the hazelnuts, Erythritol, cocoa powder and vanilla extract in a food processor. Now pour in the mixture from step 1 and blend again.

3. Place mixture in freezer for 10 minutes. Make 10 balls from the mixture with your hands by rolling each ball around a whole hazelnut so it sits in the middle of the mixture.

4. Roll each ball into the chopped whole nuts and hazelnuts until fully covered. Serve immediately!

Calories: 145 Carbs: 2.4g Fat: 14g Protein: 1.9g Fiber: 1.7g

Blueberry Fat Bombs

Ingredients (serves 12)

¾ cup of cream cheese
½ cup blueberries
5 tablespoons butter
¼ tsp vanilla extract
3 tablespoons coconut oil
1/8 tsp sea salt

Instructions

1. Blend all the ingredients together in a food blender until smooth.

2. Spoon the mixture evenly into a parchment-lined loaf pan.

3. Freeze mixture for 1 hour until firm. Remove and cut into 12 pieces.

4. Return to freezer for another hour until mixture is solid. Remove from pan then serve!

Calories: 115 Carbs: 1g Fat: 12g Protein: 1g Fiber: 1.2g

CHOCOLATE TAHINI FAT BOMBS

Ingredients (serves 16)

2 ounces cacao butter
1 ounce cacao baking chocolate
¼ cup coconut oil
¼ cup Swerve
½ cup tahini
Flaky sea salt

Instructions

1. Melt together the coconut oil, baking chocolate and cacao butter in a small saucepan on a low heat. Stir while heating.

2. Whisk in the Swerve and tahini with the above mixture until fully combined.

3. Line a muffin tin with liners and scoop the mixture into each compartment.

4. Chill for 30 minutes before serving.

Calories: 125 Carbs: 1g Fat: 12g Protein:

THANK YOU ONCE AGAIN!

Thank you once again for your purchase of The Keto Bread Cookbook 2019! As a one-man (woman) operation, I strive to put ALL my effort into producing high quality information – but please forgive me for any slight grammar errors you may have encountered!

Much love,

Megan

CPSIA information can be obtained
at www.ICGtesting.com
Printed in the USA
LVHW082352050619
620330LV00030B/914/P